Javier Díez Chamarro
Alejandro Barranco López

Geometric model predictor of dose in organs at risk

Javier Díez Chamarro
Alejandro Barranco López

Geometric model predictor of dose in organs at risk

in breast treatment with tangential beam external beam radiation therapy

ScienciaScripts

Cover image: www.ingimage.com

This book is a translation from the original published under ISBN 978-3-8417-6269-6.

Publisher:
Sciencia Scripts
is a trademark of
Dodo Books Indian Ocean Ltd. and OmniScriptum S.R.L publishing group

120 High Road, East Finchley, London, N2 9ED, United Kingdom
Str. Armeneasca 28/1, office 1, Chisinau MD-2012, Republic of Moldova, Europe
Printed at: see last page
ISBN: 978-620-5-66508-4

Contents

Acknowledgements

Art is I, science is we.

- Claude Bernard, An Introduction to the Study of Experimental Medicine, Claude Bernard, An Introduction to the Study of Experimental Medicine.

This work not only puts an end to the Master in Medical Physics, but also serves as a closure to my residency in Hospital Radiophysics at the Hospital Clinico Universitario Lozano Blesa in Zaragoza.

I would like to thank, in black and white, the partners of my formation in the application of physics to health during these years, between 2018 and 2021.

First of all, I am forever grateful to the colleagues of the Physics and Radiological Protection Service of the Lozano Blesa, for riding on the shoulders of great people and colleagues. Thanks to Esther, Araceli, Miguel, Alejandro Gartia, Sheila, Sonia, Javier Jimenez, Pedro, Pablo, Mamen, Marta, Aurora, Carlos, Luis David, Bea, Evangelina, Yolanda, Celia.

Special mention to Alejandro Barranco, creator of the idea and promoter, collaborator and tutor of this work. Also, partner of multiple compilers. Thanks for your contributions, advice, conversations, ideas, discussions and revisions.

Thanks also to all the members of the Radiotherapy Service of the same hospital, from the first to the last, with whom I have shared enriching experiences and learned in all facets about the complex and hard, but at the same time rewarding, work behind the application of radiation to the treatment of cancer.

On the other hand, thanks to Cristina Santa Marta, also tutor of this work and coordinator of the Master in Medical Physics, for always being so quick and efficient, either by phone, email or videoconference, responding to reviews, doubts and solving a wide range of bureaucratic problems throughout the Master. In this sense, thanks also to Asuncion Gonzalez and Maria Belen Gallardo, for having managed to enrol me against the clock and successfully in all the subjects in each of the courses.

In addition, and as always in every step I take, I would like to thank those who from the first day of my life have supported my training: thank you dad and mum. I am always indebted to you.

Summary

This paper presents a model based on patient anatomy to predict the percentage of ipsilateral lung and/or heart volume receiving at least a certain dose in breast treatments with static tangential external beam radiation therapy fields.

The model is based on a correlation between the percentage of healthy organ that is directly irradiated by the tangential beam and the predicted variable mentioned above: percentage of healthy organ that receives at least a certain dose.

One of the keys to the model is to calculate the first variable, percentage of healthy organ that is directly irradiated by the tangential beam, from the DICOM structure file of each patient.

The prediction is made from this variable, computed by a programme that has been developed for this purpose, and from the equation of the correlation line of the dose to be predicted. To obtain the slope and the ordinate at the origin, it is necessary to calibrate the model on the basis of treatments already planned, whose distribution of absorbed dose in the organs of interest is known.

Two independent models have been calibrated (correlation lines obtained) by disease laterality: right lung in exclusive right breast irradiation and left lung and heart on the left.

Both models show good correlation in the dose range between 20 and 90% of the prescribed dose to the affected breast and exceptionally good correlation between 35 and 85%.

To *my father, Antonio Diez Lopez, because a big part of you lives in me. Thank you dad, for everything. To my mother, Pepa Chamarro Salvachua, may your joy continue to shine on us.*

To Ana, because the future is ours.

Chapter 1
Introduction

The ability to understand something before it's observed is at the heart of scientific thinking.

- Carlo Rovelli, The Order Of Time

This chapter aims to contextualise the reader on: breast cancer and the role that EBRT (External Radiotherapy) plays in its treatment (section 1.1. 1.1)the equipment and techniques used (section 1.2). 1.2) and the workflow involved in an EBRT treatment (section 1.3). 1.3).
This background information is convenient for the following chapters where related topics are discussed. The reader familiar with the breast cancer TEN process can go directly to the next chapter where the objectives of this work are described.

1.1 Breast cancer and external radiotherapy

Breast cancer is the most frequent and deadliest cancer in women worldwide [1]. REDECAN (Red Espanola de Registros de Cancer) estimates that in 2021 more than 33,000 women were diagnosed with this disease [2].
Detection by mammography-based screening programmes can detect the disease at an early stage and significantly reduce mortality [3, 4]. Other causes of detection include clinical symptoms such as palpability of the lesion, pain, bleeding, nipple discharge, erythema, breast tenderness, etc.
In 64% of detections, the disease is confined to the mammary gland, while in 28%, it is also located in one or more of the three adjacent lymph node regions: axillary, clavicular or internal mammary [5].

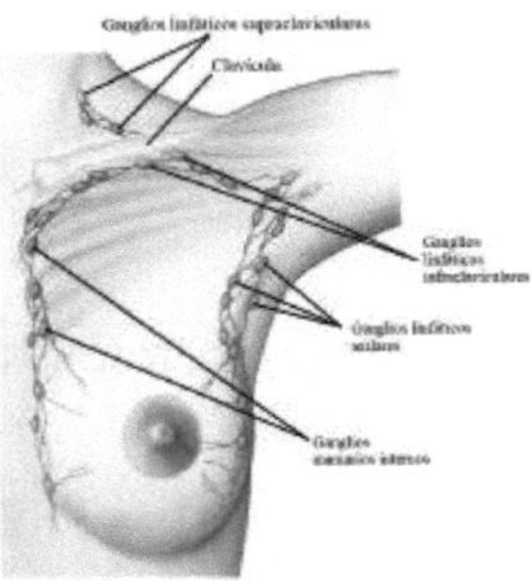

Figure 1.1: Mammary gland and adjacent lymphatic regions.

The treatment strategy in these cases where the disease has not metastasised is a primary local therapy based on surgery followed by adjuvant radiotherapy and adjuvant systemic therapy consisting of a combination of chemotherapy and radiation therapy.

and/or hormone therapy depending on the type of biomarkers [6].

The aim of post-surgery radiotherapy is to treat subclinical local disease that is unresectable in the operating theatre. Regarding the mode of radiation delivery, the most widespread division distinguishes between external beam radiation delivery or EBRT [7] and brachytherapy [8], where a radioactive source is placed inside or close to the target volume. Both can be delivered exclusively to the tumour bed, IMP (Partial Breast Irradiation), or to the whole breast (including the bed), BMI (Whole Breast Irradiation).

Radiotherapy after breast tissue-conserving surgery has been shown to be as effective as radical mastectomy in terms of local recurrence rates and survival [9]. Conservative surgery with subsequent TEN is indicated in approximately 90% of breast lumpectomies.

IMC with a dose overimpression (boost) over the operated tumour bed has demonstrated similar survival to IMC without boost but with a lower local recurrence [10] and is the standard choice of irradiation in TEN.

In addition, affected lymph node regions can be included within the volume to be irradiated in the case of positive SLNB [11] or in high-risk patients with negative SLNB [12].

1.2 LINACs for medical use and irradiation techniques

The high-energy LINAC (*Linear* Accelerator)* is the machine par excellence used in the TEN. They are often referred to simply as accelerators and are capable of delivering treatments for a wide variety of pathologies. Figure 1.2 1.2 shows some of their general parts.

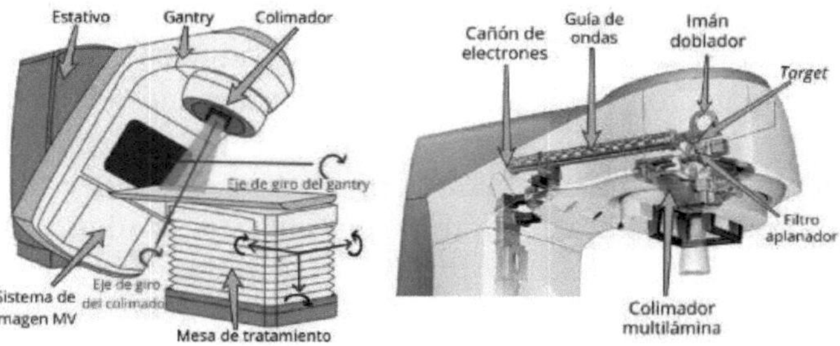

Figure 1.2: On the left, sketch of a medical accelerator and treatment table with its movements: *gantry* rotation, collimator and translations and possible rotations of the table top. On the right, detailed diagram of the ionising radiation generator and collimator system of an ONCOR accelerator, adapted image, courtesy of *Siemens Healthineers.*

These devices emit ionising radiation in the form of photons or electrons. The generation system is based on the acceleration of electrons within a waveguide with a potential difference generally ranging from 6 MV (Megavolt) to 25 MV and produces a useful beam of electrons.

For the emission of photons, a metal target is interposed on which the beam is collided. The deceleration of electrons produces by the *Bremsstrahlung* effect a photon beam with a characteristic energy spectrum which is limited by the acceleration potential. In practice, the energy of the photon beam is characterised by the potential at which the electrons are accelerated in the waveguide. Thus, the most common photon energies available in commercial medical accelerators are said to be 6, 10 or 15 MV.

*In the radiotherapeutic field, the energy of a particle is considered high when it is of the order of MeV (Megaelectron volt) or higher.

The most widespread radiation collimation system is the one based on MLC (Multileaf Collimator).Colimador *collimator*). It consists of a series of lamellae of about 10 cm in thickness and a width of a few mm. The thickness of the lamella is relevant to the beam attenuation, while the width is related to the collimation resolution, the smaller the width, the higher the resolution. The lamellae are arranged in such a way as to minimise the transmission of radiation between them. Each lamella, by means of mechanical systems, has the capacity to move unidimensionally and slide over the two adjacent lamellae. This system is mounted on the head of the accelerator and rotates in a solid manner as the collimator rotates.
This system allows the segmentation, from each *gantry* angle, of a radiation field through which it is possible to irradiate the PTV *Planning Target Volume) and protect the*(Volumen Planning Target Volume (PTV) and to protect the OAR (*Organ At* Risk) (figure 1.3). 1.3).
From the least to the most complex and technologically demanding, the following three internationally widespread techniques for the radiation treatment of TEN are distinguished.

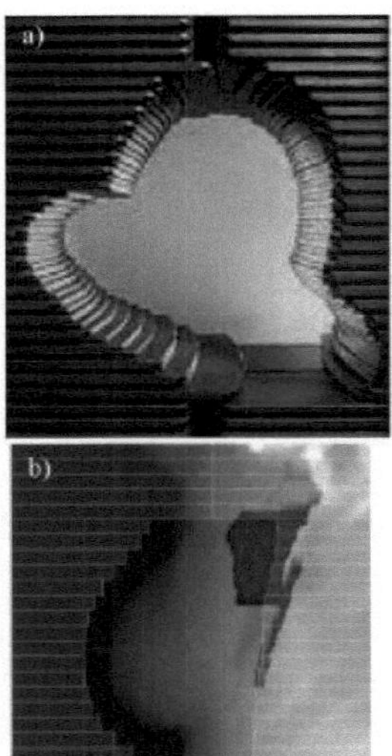

Figure 1.3: a) Frontal photograph of an MLC forming an arbitrary segment, obtained from [13]. b) BEV (*Beam Eye* View) of an anterior tangential field of an MLC conformal breast treatment. Each semi-solid rectangle represents a slice of the collimator. As seen in the RDR

(Reconstructed Digital Radiography) they all form a segment containing the projection of the affected breast at that *gantry* angle. Retrieved from [14].

- 3D-CRT (*3D* Conformal *Radiation Therapy*): This is the static treatment par excellence. In it, all geometrical and dosimetric parameters are constant during irradiation: *gantry* and collimator angle, slice positions, as well as dose rate.

- IMRT (Intensity *Modulated Radiation Therapy*): In this treatment, in each field the *gantry* and collimator rotation remain constant as well, but during irradiation the blades move modulating in each incidence orientation the integrated flux of ionising particles emerging from the head. The rate may or may not be constant depending on the LINAC model.

- VMAT (Volumetric *Modulated Arc Therapy*): This is the most dynamic treatment: during irradiation of the patient the *gantry* rotates around the patient describing a circumferential arc. In the meantime, the position of the blades and the dose rate vary in favour of an optimal treatment.

The superficial location of the breast makes the 3D-CRT treatment approach, for most patients, dosimetrically better for proximal healthy organs: ipsilateral lung, contralateral breast, contralateral lung and heart [15]. In addition, the use of this technique requires less human resources (time for treatment plan development and quality control) and technical resources (accelerator time for treatment quality control).
However, in certain cases, the geometry of the affected breast and nearby healthy organs makes it optimal for these latter seconds to use other more complex techniques, such as IMRT or VMAT.

1.3 Workflow in external radiotherapy

The radiotherapy process is carried out by a multidisciplinary team comprising radiotherapy oncology and hospital radiophysics specialists, radiotherapy and dosimetry technicians, as well as graduates in nursing. The workflow involved in TEN treatment can be seen in the following diagram:

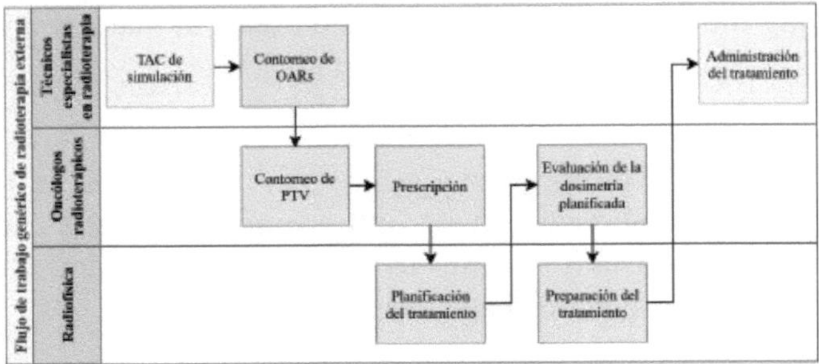

Figure 1.4: Stages and responsible parties in the generic external radiotherapy process. The ones coloured in yellow imply the presence of the patient in the hospital. Own elaboration.

Each of the stages of this general flow will be detailed below, with particular emphasis on the case of breast cancer and on the concepts of interest to this work.

Treatment simulation CT

Since the global availability of CT (Computed Tomography) and TPS (Treatment Planning System) has become more widely available. TPS Treatment Planning System(Planificacion de Tratamientos) in hospitals, external radiotherapy is not understood in hospitals, external radiotherapy cannot be understood if it is not linked to a CT (Computerised Axial Tomography) simulation image. It is called as such^ because it is used to simulate the radiotherapy treatment for each patient, optimising and calculating the dose deposited at each point in space.

This approach involves making the key double assumption of external beam therapy: at each treatment session, the patient will be placed in the same position as on the day of the mock CT (on which the treatment is planned) and will remain in the same position for the duration of the treatment.

CT scans used in radiotherapy departments are not very different from those used in diagnostic radiology. In general, they have a larger calibre than the latter, which is useful for patient restraint systems to be able to pass widely through the CT bore. Another difference is the existence of laser systems mounted on the walls and/or ceiling of the room. Each projects a cross on the opposite wall whose centre coincides with the centres of the other crosses at the same point in the room. The RTE treatment rooms with high energy LINAC have the same laser system that allows the reproducibility of the positioning. TAC TAC-accelerator positioning.

The radiation oncologist indicates the body region to be scanned and the patient's position (supine/prone). The reconstruction of the CT image results in a set of n_z axial slices with a slice thickness that, in the field of radiotherapy, is usually between 1 and 5 mm. Each of these slices has a number (nx and n_y respectively in the transverse and anteroposterior directions) of fixed pixel sizes for each x- and y-direction. The reconstruction generates nx^ny-nz voxels, each of them with a grey value whose depth has 2^{nbits} levels. All this information from the TC together with other metadata or attributes are stored digitally in files that follow the DICOM (Digital Imaging and Communications in Medicine) standard [16].

In breast irradiation treatments, generally 3 or 5 mm cut thicknesses are used in the reconstruction and the acquisition is performed craniocaudally from the base of the chin to the complete inclusion of the lungs. Positioning is mainly in the supine position using an inclined plane on which the patient's back rests as an immobiliser in order to separate the breast tissue from the clavicular region.

In specific cases of IM (left breast), the dosimetric benefit of healthy tissue in prone positioning has been demonstrated [17, 18], especially in pendulous breasts. Another technique with the same rationale (moving healthy tissue away from the target volume) is the irradiation at DIBH (Deep Inspiration Breath Hold) [19], although it is not applicable to all patients as it requires their cooperation in controlling their respiratory cycle and being able to keep it contained over time. Currently the practical implementation of these techniques is not widely used internationally and the benefits between one or the other are still a matter of debate [20].

An important task in the simulation stage is the determination of the three-dimensional coordinate origin in the image. For this purpose, the scan is carried out by attaching three metal pellets on the patient, exactly on the skin, in the centre of the cross projected from each laser (side walls and ceiling). These pellets are used because they are clearly visualised in the reconstructed image and thus the point of contact between the laser cross and the skin can be identified on the image. The origin of coordinates is established in the 3D image as the point in the axial plane where the three pellets are displayed simultaneously and where the line passing through the two lateral pellets and a perpendicular line passing through the third one intersect. In the place where they are in contact with the patient's skin, small marks are tattooed, which are useful for reproducing the CT position in the treatment room, using the same laser system.

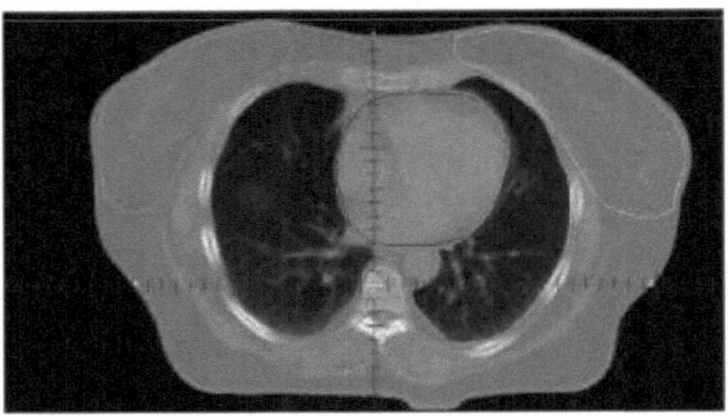

Figure 1.5: XiO planner image showing the axial slice containing the three pellets attached to the patient's skin, useful to indicate on the image the position of the origin of coordinates. CT, marked with a yellow crosshair.

Outline of structures: PTV and OAR

Once a patient image has been acquired, the need arises to segment regions of special interest. As a solution to this problem, the file was born DICOM FILE structure file was born as a solution to this problem. In this file, the information referring to these regions is encoded and is always associated to another DICOM file. DICOM FILE file containing the image information.

Each structure k is defined in this standard as an ordered set of nk three-dimensional coordinates (xi, yi, zi), with i=1, 2, ..., nk with respect to the origin. TAC of simulation.

Structure generation systems are generally based on computer programmes with tools to delimit, slice by slice and one by one, the structures of interest. Recently, solutions with automatic systems based on anatomical atlases [21, 22] or artificial intelligence [23] have been incorporated in the market to auto-segment the structures of interest. OAR. However, in such cases it is advisable to have these structures reviewed and edited manually, if necessary, by a specialist.

In either generation method, the end result is a set of ROIs (Regions

Of Interest). Each structure is encoded by a set of kz sequences. Each sequence is defined on an axial plane and has the associated z-axis coordinate of the plane to which it belongs. A sequence is composed of one or more series of ordered two-dimensional points represented by coordinates in the x-y plane. These points are considered in planning systems and other structure viewers. DICOM structure viewers as vertices of polygons. A wide variety of algebraic and geometric operations can be visualised and performed through the computer tools incorporated in each programme, as well as interpolating or extrapolating points in planes where they have not been contoured if necessary.

It is worth noting two types of structures, the PTV and the OAR. A PTV, as its name suggests, is a volume to be irradiated. The lesion or lesions to be treated are contained in this volume. In contrast, the OAR are all those organs which, as a collateral effect of the treatment, will receive a certain dose that must be monitored, optimised and/or limited.

In the case of this work, the fundamental ROIs are: PTV of the affected breast, ipsilateral lung, contralateral breast and heart.

Prescription and restrictions

The radiation oncologist is responsible for prescribing the dose administration. He/she must prescribe to each PTV a PD (Dose de Prescription) and indicate a fractionation or number of sessions in which this total dose is administered. Equivalently, you can indicate the dose per session in addition to the PD. Finally, indicate the treatment schedule and its frequency, i.e. schedule which day or days the treatment will be given and how many times per day.

Standard treatments are scheduled once a day, five days a week: Monday to Friday. The prescribed dosage depends on the pathology, with the standard dosage per session at TEN is 2 Gy.

In addition to the prescription, fractionation and frequency, the radiation oncologist indicates dose coverage criteria on the PTV and dose constraints for OAR that the planned treatment must comply with.

The criteria shall be expressed with the following score:

$$V_i(D)[\%] > o < \% \text{ volumen de } i$$

where V_i (D) [%] is the percentage of the volume of structure i that receives at least one dose D, which must be (as indicated by the target or constraint) greater or less than a certain volume of structure i. The dose D is expressed as a percentage of the prescription dose. In addition, it is common to limit the maximum dose of a structure or its average dose Dmed .
The PTV coverage criteria commonly used in standard treatments are based on the document [24] and are as follows:

- V_{PTV} (95%) > 95%
- V_{PTV} (107%) < 1% V (107%) < 1% V (107%) < 1% V

That is, at least 95 % of the PTV has a dose higher than 95 % of the prescribed dose and at most 1 % of the PTV volume has a dose higher than 107 % of the PD.
The dose tolerance of each organ at risk depends on the fractionation of the treatment, and therefore, so do the restrictions imposed. Table 1.1 lists, according to the literature, some of the different whole breast TEN treatment schedules and their restrictions.
Fractionation into BMI has a historical trend towards hypofractionation. Follow-up of the START clinical trial [25] demonstrates that moving from a standard fractionation of 2 Gy per session over 25 sessions (50 Gy total) to 2.67 Gy per session over 15 sessions (40.05 Gy total) is safe and effective. It is currently the most common fractionation. A more extreme hypofractionation, favoured in the wake of the outbreak of the *COVID-19* pandemic worldwide, is the one reported under the *FAST* and *FAST-Forward* clinical trials, respectively [26] and [27], in which treatment is delivered in 5 sessions with a PD of 26 or 27 Gy (5.2 or 5.4 Gy/fraction).
The affected lymph node volumes are treated with the same dose and fractionation as the breast. In indicated cases, an extra dose is given to a VTP inside the breast VTP containing the tumour bed, which reduces the risk of local recurrence as opposed to increased toxicity in the breast. This over-impression of dose is called *boost*. The total prescribed dose to the tumour bed is 48 Gy in moderate fractionation and 29 Gy in extreme fractionation. These doses already include that the breast receives 40.05 or 26/27 Gy, i.e. the dose overimpression respectively is: 7.95 Gy (in 15 fractions) and 3/2 Gy (in 5 fractions).

Radiotherapy treatment planning

At this stage the radiophysicist is responsible for a triple task:

- Define the necessary instructions that the LINAC must be able to reproduce in the administration of the treatment.

- Such instructions or treatment plan should be such as to produce a dose distribution over the CT scan that complies, to the best extent possible, with the coverage and restrictions indicated by the radiation oncologist.

- That the computed dose distribution is faithful to that which will actually be deposited. This includes checking that the initial reference state and subsequent quality controls of each equipment involved in the process (simulation CT [28], TPS [29], LINAC and detectors used [30]) are correct.

TPS are software programmes that assist in this task. They employ dose calculation algorithms configured on the basis of experimental measurements for each LINAC [31]. Once a treatment plan is created, the programme computes the dose distribution associated with irradiating it on the patient. This distribution is a volumetric dose matrix whose resolution in standard treatments is 3 x 3 x 3 mm in each dimension, i.e. each voxel of this size is assigned a unique value of average absolute dose absorbed by the tissue that contains it. This dosimetric information is stored in the DICOM FILE dose file.
TPS are able to generate files DICOM FILES files containing the necessary instructions for the accelerator to radiate the treatment in a way that reproduces on the patient the dose distribution computed on the CT. These files consist of a series of checkpoints or discretisations of the treatment. At each checkpoint, among other parameters, the following are specified:

- Beam energy.
- Angle of rotation of the collimator.
- Gantry pivoting position.
- Position of each of the MLC blades.
- UM (Monitor Unit)† to radiate.

The following figure shows images from a commercial TPS where we

†The UMs are a quantisation of the radiation generated inside the accelerator head. This is indirectly detected by a redundant system of calibrated ionisation chambers which cut off the trigger when any one of them reaches the planned value.

can observe as an illustrative example VMAT and 3D tangential conformal planning of an MI irradiation, as well as isodose curves relative to the PD in an axial slice of the CT:

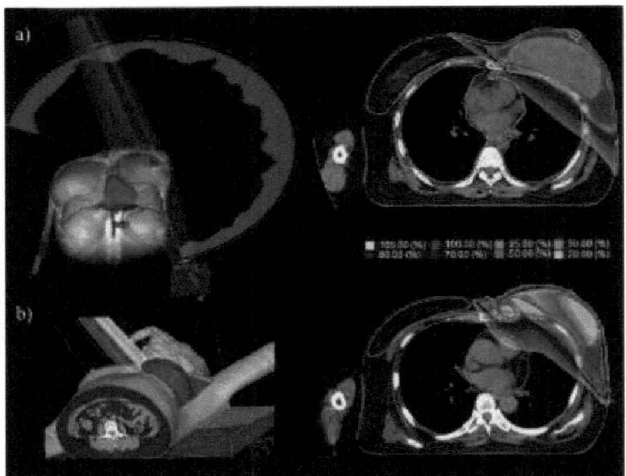

Figure 1.6: Rendered images of MI treatments with techniques: a) VMAT and b) 3D conformal tangential. Respectively on the right, dose distributions of an axial slice of the planning CT. Adapted image, obtained from [32].

Table 1.1: Full breast irradiation schedules with TEN with indications, prescriptions, fractionations and restrictions.

TEN in breast cancer					
Treatment scheme	**Indication**	**Technique**	**Dose (Gy)**	**Fractions**	**Restrictions**
Moderately hypofractionated [ ]	After conservative surgery 0 mastectomy	3D-CRT IMRT VMAT	40.05 Gy to breast/wall, involved lymph node areas and, if indicated, 48 Gy simultaneous in bed	15x(2.67 Gy breast/wall, affected lymph node areas and, if indicated, 3.2 Gy tumour bed) 1 fx/day, 15 days, 3 weeks	Pip: V(12 Gy)<15% V(12 Gy)<15% V(12 Gy)<15% V(12 Gy)<15 Cor: V(2Gy)<30%, V(10Gy)<5%.
Fast Forward [ ]	After conservative surgery 0 mastectomy	3D-CRT IMRT VMAT	26 Gy to breast/wall, affected lymph node areas and, if indicated, 29 Gy simultaneo	5x(5.2 Gy breast/wall, affected lymph node areas and, if	Pip: V(8 Gy)<15% Cor: V(1.5 Gy)<30%, V(7 Gy) <5%.

			us to bedside	indicated, 5.8 tumour bed) 1 fx/day, 5 days, 1 week	
Hypofractionated weekly 3.]	After conservative surgery 0 mastectomy	3D-CRT IMRT VMAT	30 Gy breast/wall, 27.5 Gy affected lymph node areas and, if indicated, 42 Gy breast/wall, 27.5 Gy affected lymph node areas and, if indicated, 42 Gy bed	5x(6 Gy breast/wall y 5.5 Gy affected lymph node areas) and, if indicated, 2x6 Gy tumour bed) 1 fx/week, 5-7 days, 5-7 weeks	Pip: V(20 Gy)<45%, V(30 Gy)<35% Cor: V(5 Gy)<40% Cor: V(5 Gy)<40% Cor: V(5 Gy)<40 V(20 Gy)<20% MC: V(5 Gy)<15% V(5 Gy)<15% V(5 Gy)<15% V(5 Gy)<15
Moderate preoperative	Preoperative RT	3D-CRT IMRT	40.05 Gy to	15x(2.67 Gy	Pip: V(12 Gy)<15%

hypofractionated [J4].	with QT (HER2+) 0 with HT in luminal	VMAT	breast/wall, involved lymph node areas and, if indicated, 48 Gy simultaneous in bed	breast/wall, involved lymph node areas and, if indicated, 3.2 Gy tumour bed) 1 fx/day, 15 days, 3 weeks	V(12 Gy)<15% V(12 Gy)<15% V(12 Gy)<15 Cor: V(2 Gy)<30% V(2 Gy)<30% V(2 Gy)<30% V(2 Gy)<30 V(10 Gy)<5% V(10 Gy)<5% V(10 Gy)<5% V(10 Gy)<5

Volume dose histogram

In addition to the spatial representation of the dose distribution, the planners represent the so-called DVH *Dose Volume* (Histogram Dosis Volumen)is a graph comprising a series of curves useful for a compact evaluation of the dose distribution of a planner. It is a cumulative dose histogram that is calculated for each structure contoured in the treatment from the DICOM FILES dose and structure files. Each structure has an associated cumulative dose-volume curve. The x-axis represents the dose, expressed either in absolute units (usually cGy) or as a percentage relative to the PD of the treatment. The y-axis represents the volume of the structure receiving at least a certain dose D(x), usually expressed as a percentage of the volume relative to the structure or in cubic centimetres. The figure 1.7 shows an example of a DVH comparison.

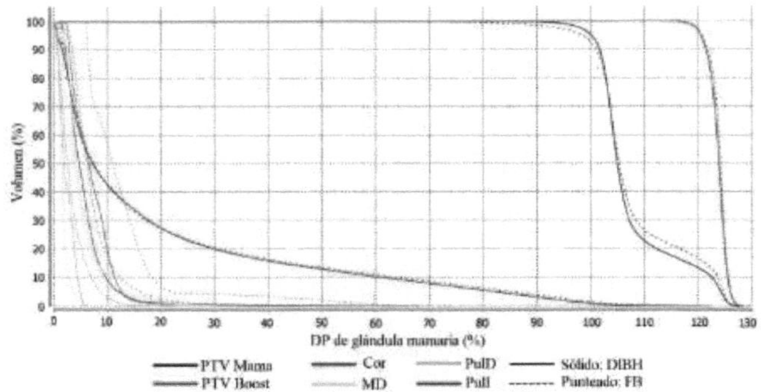

Figure 1.7: DVH in relative units comparing a left breast treatment in FB *(Free Breathing)* vs. another in DIBH. Image adapted for academic purposes from [35].

The DVH allows a quick assessment of whether the dosimetry meets the imposed constraints as these are representable as points on the histogram. For example, in the DVH in figure 1.7, the left lung volume receiving at least 30% of the prescription dose is 20%, which does not meet the restriction imposed for moderate hypofractionated treatment in table 1.1, V(30%)<15%.

Evaluation of planned dosimetry

In this task, the radiation oncologist checks that the dose distribution proposed in the planning is clinically acceptable and, if so, approves the treatment. If this is not the case, the treatment must be re-planned.

Treatment preparation

This stage includes the associated tasks for the LINAC can deliver the treatment and ensure that each irradiated session is properly recorded. It may also include verification of the plan [36], either with redundant dose distribution calculation software tools or by irradiation of the planned accelerator treatment on suitable detectors with subsequent analysis. If there is a significant disparity between the planned and the result of the verification, it is advisable to investigate the reason and/or re-plan.

Treatment management

In general, each treatment session consists of two parts:

- **Patient positioning**: In the CT treatment simulation, a patient position is established with respect to the treatment machine. Before starting treatment, it is essential that the patient is positioned in this position in accordance with the planned treatment simulation. For this purpose, most commercial LINACs include integrated kV or MV X-ray imaging systems or both, with which you can optionally perform IGRT (Image , prior to treatment.Radiotherapy Guided por) prior to treatment. IGRT consists of acquiring an image of the patient in the treatment position, subsequently the image obtained is registered with the reference image (planning CT or RDR obtained from it), obtaining a series of translations and optionally rotations to bring the real position of the patient to the reference position.

- **Treatment irradiation**: Once the patient is in the appropriate position, the treatment is irradiated. During irradiation, the patient is monitored by video and audio systems by radiotherapy specialists. They are responsible for ensuring that the treatment is delivered as planned and can pause and resume treatment if necessary.

Chapter 2

Objectives

It is wrong to think that the task of physics is to find out how Nature is. Physics concerns what we say about Nature.

- Niels Bohr, On Quantum Physics

The aim of this work is to predict which is the most suitable technique for radiotherapy treatment of breast cancer. Specifically, it aims to predict whether treatment with tangential 3D-CRT is suitable or whether a more complex technique should be used.
For this purpose, the percentage of OAR absorbing a dose capable of producing adverse effects will be calculated if treatment is planned with 3D-CRT. 3D-CRT TECHNIQUE. If the percentage of OAR is higher than the imposed restrictions, it would be advisable to plan the treatment with a more complex technique.
In order to calculate the percentage of the RAO that would receive a dose D indicative of possible adverse effects, a new geometric parameter will be defined, which we will call the volume of exposed RAO. This parameter depends on the anatomical characteristics of each patient and will be correlated with the volume of OAR absorbing this dose D. This correlation will assist in the choice of the treatment technique to be used.
A theoretical model and an algorithm will be developed that, according to the rules of the model, will obtain the correlation lines between the volume of OAR absorbing a dose D and the volume of OAR exposed. Since the organs at risk are different for left and right breast treatments, a model will be made for each case. Models will be calibrated from existing schedules for a range of D doses covering a wide range.

Chapter 3
Methods

What we often forget is that a model is not a description of reality; it is a description of our assumptions about reality.

- Jeremy Gunawardena, Models in biology: 'accurate descriptions of our pathetic thinking'.

3.1 The theoretical framework

The basis of the model is the correlation between the following two variables:

- The **percentage of OAR intersected by the optimal beam**. This is a purely geometric variable that depends on the anatomy of each patient and is computed from the contoured structures on the planning CT according to the rules described below. It is denoted for each organ at risk i as VI_i (Volume Intersected of organ i)where i=Cor (Heart), PulD (Right Lung) or PulI (Left Lung). It is expressed as a percentage of the total volume of organ i.

- The **percentage of OAR receiving at least one dose** D. The dose is expressed as a percentage with respect to the PD of the PTV: D[%]. For each structure i this variable is denoted as Vi (D[%])[%]. This will be the predicted target magnitude.

Initially, it is necessary to calibrate the model on the basis of the plans already made, whose Vi(D[%])[%] values are known (from the DVH curve of each structure). To obtain the slope m and the ordinate at the origin n of the correlation line, a least squares adjustment of the data is performed. VIi[%] - *Vi* (D[%])[%] to a straight line. As a measure of the degree of correlation between these values, the Pearson correlation coefficient r, the square root of the R2 statistic that measures the goodness of fit of linear regression, is used.
Once m(D) and n(D) have been determined, it is necessary to compute the VIi to make the prediction of Vi(D), as follows:

$$V_i(D)^{Predicho} = m(D) \cdot VI_i + n(D) \tag{3.1}$$

Computation of *VIi[%]*

The starting point of the model are three-dimensional structures contoured on the planning CT. Each treatment will be considered as a geometrical system consisting of the following structures:

- PTV of the affected breast
- MC (Contralateral Breast)
- PulI
- PulD
- Cor

In MD (Right Breast) treatments, VI_{PulD}[%] is computed, whereas in MI *VIPulI* [%] and *VICor* [%]. These volumes are intended to estimate in each case the intersection between the OAR and the optimal direct beam and are defined as follows (visual interpretation in figure 3.1):

$$VI_{PulD} = \sum_j \Delta z \left([PulD]_j \bigcap [H_{az}(\theta_{opt})]_j \right) \quad (3.2)$$

$$VI_{PulI} = \sum_j \Delta z \left([PulI]_j \bigcap [H_{az}(\theta_{opt})]_j \right) \quad (3.3)$$

$$VI_{Cor} = \sum_j \Delta z \left([Cor]_j \bigcap [H_{az}(\theta_{opt})]_j \right) \quad (3.4)$$

where:

- The summation $\sum_j$ is extended to all CT slices with *j* referring to the jth slice.

- Δz is the CT slice thickness or distance between two axial images‡ . It is a characteristic value of the reconstructed image.

- $[PulD]_j$, $[PulI]_j$ and $[Cor]_j$ are respectively the right lung, left lung and heart structures outlined on slice j .

- $[H_{az}(\theta_{opt})]_j$ is the representation of the optimal treatment beam on slice j of the reconstruction. This structure is modelled according to the rules written in the next section.

‡The n images of the reconstruction

Beam modelling $[\mathrm{Haz}(\theta)]$

It is intended to delimit the direct beam which, after being collimated by the MLCirradiates the breast. For this purpose, the structure $[\mathrm{Haz}(\theta)]$ will be created, defined as a series of rectangles in the axial slices where there are PTV breast. These rectangles have a series of common characteristics:

- They contain the entire PTV, being tangent to it on its posterior contour.

- The angle of incidence θ (represents the *gantry* angle) is the inclination of the major sides of the rectangle with the anteroposterior axis of the patient. It is the same for all slices.

- The larger side of the rectangle overlapping the patient must go all the way through the patient. That is, no corner of the rectangle should be inside the patient.

3.1.1 Optimal angle of tangential irradiance

The optimum angle of tangential irradiation 0_{opt} is defined as such that the intersection between the three-dimensional beam [Beam(0_{opt})] and the structures [Cor] and [PIp (Pulmon Ipsilateral)] is minimal and does not intersect the [MC] by more than 2% of its total volume:

$$\theta_{opt} = \theta \mid \min\left\{[\mathrm{Haz}(\theta)]\bigcap[\mathrm{PIp}] + [\mathrm{Haz}(\theta)]\bigcap[\mathrm{Cor}]\right\} \wedge [\mathrm{Haz}(\theta)]\bigcap[\mathrm{MC}] < 2\%\mathrm{Vol}([\mathrm{MC}]) \quad (3.5)$$

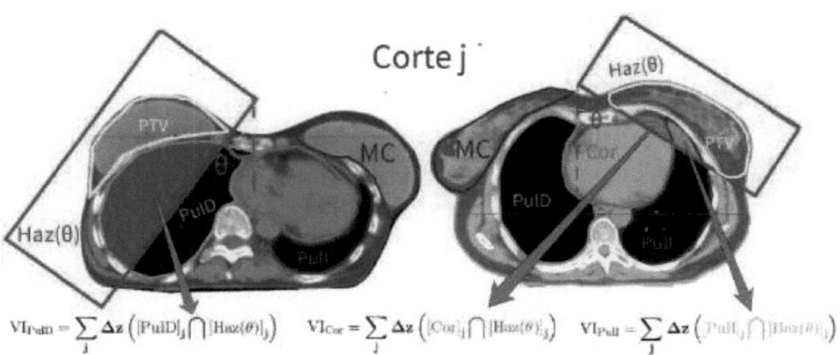

$$VI_{PulD} = \sum_j \Delta z\left([\mathrm{PulD}]_j \bigcap [\mathrm{Haz}(\theta)]_j\right) \quad VI_{Cor} = \sum_j \Delta z\left([\mathrm{Cor}]_j \bigcap [\mathrm{Haz}(\theta)]_j\right) \quad VI_{PulI} = \sum_j \Delta z\left([\mathrm{PulI}]_j \bigcap [\mathrm{Haz}(\theta)]_j\right)$$

Figura 1: Graphical representation of an arbitrary *j-slice* of the planning TAC where the structures and definitions of interest of the model are visualised. On the left an MD case and on the right an MI case. MI CASE. The case MD CASE case shows a beam incidence angle *0* far away from the optimum.

3.2 The programme

To implement the model, a code is developed in Python programming language capable of, starting from a file of structures DICOM, compute VI $_{PulD}$[%] in MD treatments or VIPulI [%] and VICor [%] in MI treatments.

In addition, in order to calibrate the model, it is able to obtain by interpolation, from files with the DVH information, the Vi (D)[%] of Cor, PulD and PulI for a series of Dj doses of interest.

Figure 3.2 shows the programme algorithm which will serve as an index to explain the details.

The program acts on a directory, configured as an internal variable in the code, which contains the files DICOM FILES structure files and the DVH text files of all patients. It is important that the names of both files of the same patient contain the same patient identification (in our case the code "AR" or health code of the Autonomous Community of Aragon) so that the program can match them. Initially, it creates a list in which each element includes patient identification information, the path to its structure file and the path to the text file DVH. The execution of the program itself is an iteration over the elements of this list. For each element it does the following:

3.2.1 Reading and identification of volumes

Using the *pydicom* library decodes and stores in variables all the information contained in the file DICOM FILE structures file. From it we obtain the following information:

- **CT reconstruction slice thickness, Az**. This value is the distance between consecutive axial slices reconstructed on the TAC simulation. This information does not appear directly in the DICOM FILE structure file but can be inferred. Assuming that contours are contoured only on reconstructed slices (and not on interpolations of these), *Sz* is obtained as the minimum non-zero difference between the longitudinal z-coordinates of the set of points constituting the structures. It is needed to calculate volumes of structures as a sum over the area of the structure in an axial slice times that slice thickness.

- **PTV breast and laterality**. The PTV breast is taken as the one with the smaller longitudinal z-coordinate (more caudal), other possible PTVs are PTV other possible PTVs present, if any, would be the *boost* and/or lymph node volumes, which in any case have minimum z-coordinates greater than that of the breast PTV due to their superior location.

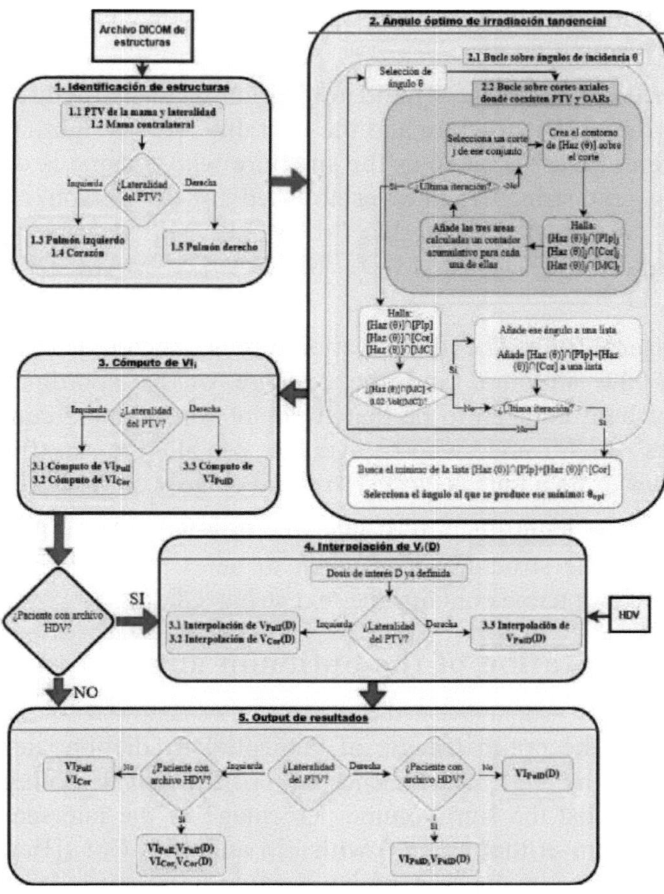

Figura 2: Flow of processes carried out by the developed code.

To do this, a first list of PTVs is made by iterating over all the structures present in the file and selecting those whose RTROIInterpretedType attribute is equal to 'PTV'. Iterating over that list, a second list is made where each item is the minimum z-coordinate of every PTV. From this second list we take as PTV the one with the lowest minimum z is taken as mother PTV.

Laterality is determined according to the sign of the average of all x-coordinates of the points composing the structure identified as PTV breast. It will be right if the sign is positive (average greater than 0) or left otherwise.

- **Contralateral breast**. The identification of this structure is based on the name of the structure and the laterality. If it is right lateral, the contralateral breast is taken as the structure whose name is one of the following text strings (names established by the person outlining): 'MAM_I , 'MAM-I', 'MAM_IZ', 'MAM _I', 'MI'. If left, any of the following: 'MAM_D', 'MAM-D', 'MAMA D', 'MAM DRCHA' or 'MAMA_D'.

- **Ipsilateral lung**. The identification of this structure is based on the name of the structure and the average of its coordinates. The ipsilateral lung is taken to be that structure whose name contains the characters 'PUL' and whose average of all the x (transverse) coordinates of its points is closest to the average x of the PTV breast.

- **Heart**. The identification of this structure is made on the basis of the name of the structure, it is taken to be Cor is taken to be the structure whose name contains the text string 'COR'.

3.2.2 Computation of the optimum angle of tangential irradiance

To calculate the optimal angle of tangential irradiation, iterate in a loop varying the angle of incidence of *0* of the *gantry,* noting in each iteration in a list the sum volume percentage of the intersection of a simulated beam at that angle 0 with PIp and with Cor ([Beam(0)] p| [PIp] + [Haz(θ)]∩[Cor]), : as long as the intersection with MC is less than 2% of its volume. To calculate this volume, at each 0 it is iterated over the TAC cuts with axial z-coordinates where coexists PTV and OAR coexist (a list of common z-coordinates is created beforehand). In each slice j , the following three processes are performed:

- **Creation of the contour [Beam(0)]**$_j$. This contour is a rectangle which fulfils the characteristics described in 3.1is defined by the coordinates of its four vertices. The following procedure is used to calculate the coordinates:

- Define a line R with slope m_R =-cot(0) passing through the point (5_{lat} 10 cm,10 cm), where:

– Se define una recta R con pendiente m_R=-cot(θ) que pasa por el punto (δ_{lat}10 cm,10 cm), donde:

$$\delta_{lat} = \begin{cases} +1 \text{ si lateralidad derecha} \\ \text{-1 si lateralidad izquierda} \end{cases} \quad (3.6)$$

The distance from that line to all the points that form the polygon of the PTV in that cut j is calculated to find the point with the smallest distance. This will be the point of the PTV that will be tangent to the side of the rectangle inside the patient.

These first two items are illustrated in figure 3.3 left.

— Based on this point and the slope of the line, the vertices of the rectangle are calculated. The vertices of the interior side are taken as those which, being on the tangent line to the PTV, are 50 cm away from the point of the PTV closest to the original line R.

— The other two vertices are taken from the two previous ones at a distance of 50 cm from each of them in a direction perpendicular to the tangent line and in an external direction to the patient.

— The final result is a rectangle of 100 x 50 cm whose major sides are inclined 0 degrees with respect to the patient's anteroposterior axis and whose inner major side is tangent to the PTV contoured in that cut at one point.

These last three items are illustrated in figure 3.3 right.

- **Calculation of the area of each OAR in that slice**. Using the functions of the *Polygon* class of the *shapely.geometry* library, the area formed by the polygon composed by the points of each OAR is calculated. OAR: PIp, Cor and MC.

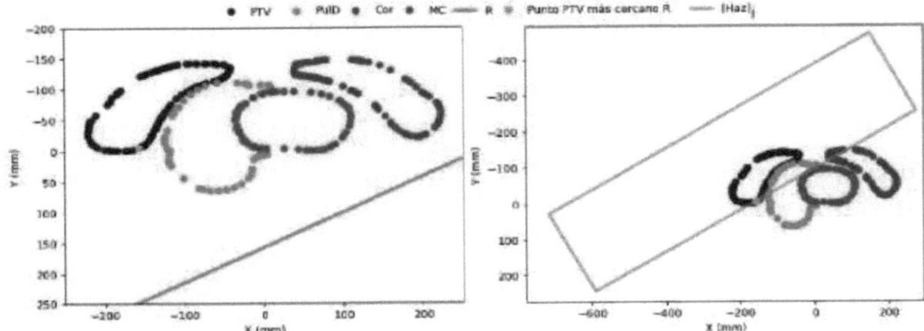

Figure 3.3: Diagram generated by the programme during the simulation of a right breast case with 0=60° at an arbitrary axial slice *j* showing: (left) sets of points of the structures of interest, the generated R line, the PTV point closest to the line; (right) set of points of the structures of interest and the [Beam (0)]j structure. In this patient 0_{opt} =42°.

- **Calculation of the exposed area in that slice**. Using also *shapely.geometry* we calculate the intersection polygon of each of the risk organs: PIp, Cor and MC and the area of each of them.

To calculate the volume of each OAR and the volume intersected by the beam of each of them, the value of the areas calculated in each slice will be stored cumulatively, multiplying by Az in each iteration to obtain these variables at the end of the loop.
If the intersected volume of MC is less than 2% of its volume, the angle of incidence 0 of the iteration is recorded in one list and the sum of the percentages of PIp and Cor in another.
When the iteration on the angles of incidence is finished, the minimum of the first list is searched and to which angle of incidence it corresponds in the second list. That will be the angle 0_{opt} , according to 3.5.

3.2.3 Computation of exposed volume of organ at risk

Once 0opt is computed, using this angle of incidence, the volume of OAR intersected by the beam is calculated for left heart and lung in case of MI and right lung in case of MD following the procedure of the previous section.

3.2.4 Interpolation of the volume of organ at risk receiving at least a certain dose

If the programme detects that a '.grf' file exists for the patient in question, it decodes that text file. The file DVH FILE file from the TPS has absolute units of dose and volume. Based on the maximum dose received, it identifies the prescription. In order to create a uniform, prescription-independent model, the DVH curves are renormalised so that 95% of the breast PTV volume has at least 95% of the PD of 4005 cGy. The identification of the structures of interest in the file is performed using the names present in the DICOM FILE. Then, with the *scipy* library, the Vi(Dj) value(s) for the desired Dj doses (entered as values in the code) are interpolated. According to the laterality i=PulD=PulD at MD and i==Cor, Pull in MI.

3.2.5 Generation of results

Using the *openpyxl* library the following data for each patient is dumped into an *Excel* file for further analysis:

- Patient ID.
- Laterality.
- Longitudinal distance between contours Az.
- Name of the structure identified as PTV.
- Volume of the structure identified as PTV according to TPS §.
- Volume of the structure identified as PTV.
- Name of the structure identified as PIp.
- Volume of the structure identified as PIp according to TPS.
- Volume of the structure identified as PIp.
- Name of the structure identified as Cor.
- Volume of the structure identified as Cor according to TPS.
- Volume of the structure identified as Cor.
- Name of the structure identified as MC.

§The volumes of the TPS structures may differ from those calculated by the programme because they are computed differently. The programme obtains this value for each organ at risk from the DVH, according to Vi(D=0 Gy) [cm^3] volume of OAR i receiving at least 0 Gy.

- Volume of the structure identified as MC according to TPS.
- Volume of the structure identified as MC.
- Optimum angle of irradiation θ_{opt} .
- VIPIp[%].
- VP Ip(Dj)[%] (if file DVH FILE file exists).
- VICor [%] (if left lateral).
- VCor (Dj)[%] (if left laterality and if archive DVH FILE file exists).

3.3 Model calibration

Two independent models are developed: MD and MI. In both cases, the doses Dj (expressed as a percentage with respect to the PD) for which V $_{OAR}$(Dj)[%] will be predicted are:

$$D_j[\%] = j \cdot 2.5\% \text{ con } j = 1, 2, ..., 39 \quad (3.7)$$

Patient selection

A cross-sectional cohort of 96 patients diagnosed with early-stage breast cancer who have received TEN exclusively in one mammary gland (57 on the right and 37 on the left) or costal wall (2 cases of MD) between 2020 and 2021 at the Hospital Clmico Universitario Lozano Blesa in Zaragoza.
In 86% of cases (54 MD and 29 IM) the tumour bed was irradiated with a higher dose than the rest of the breast. In the remaining 14% (5 cases of MD and 8 of MI), the whole breast/costal wall was irradiated homogeneously.

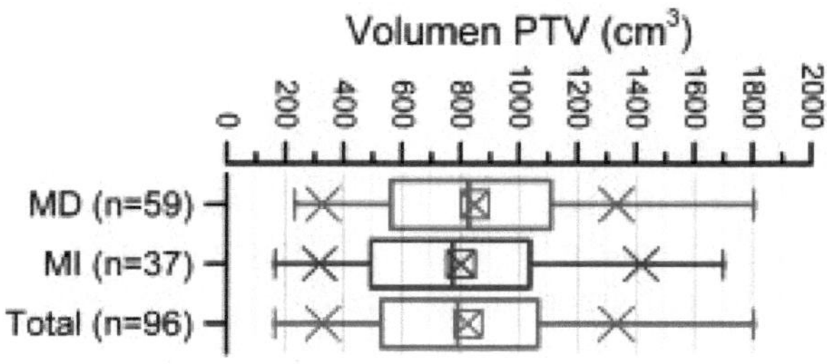

Figure 3.4: Box plot of the irra- diated volume. - indicates minimum and maximum, x 10th and 90th percentiles, ^ average. The horizontal lines in the box indicate quartile 1, median or quartile 2 and quartile 3.

Simulation and contouring

All images acquired for treatment simulation were obtained on a General Electric HiSpeed NX/i CT scanner. All patients were positioned supine, head first. The slice thickness of the reconstruction was 5 mm in all cases, except for 1 MD and 2 MI which were done with 3 mm. An inclined plane was used for immobilisation. The structures were contoured with the TPS *PCRT 3D* tools of *Tecnicas Radioflsicas S.L.* The lungs were contoured using the segmentation tool based on the grey level. Contralateral breast and heart are contoured manually by a radiotherapy and dosimetry technician. The breast PTV is manually contoured by the radiation oncologist according to international consensus guidelines [37, 38]. Figure 3.4 3.4 depicts the PTV volume distributions of the patients in each model and the total. All structures are contoured exclusively on the CT slices of the reconstruction.

Prescription and restrictions

The prescriptions in a total of 39 patients (24 MD and 15 MI) was 4005 cGy in the mammary gland in 15 sessions (267 cGy/fraction) and in the case of the presence of *boost* (20 cases of MD and 7 of MI) was prescribed in an integrated manner with 4800 cGy (320 cGy/fraction).
56 patients (34 MD and 22 MI) were given a treatment schedule of 2600 cGy in 5 sessions (520 cGy/fraction) with an integrated dose prescription of 2900 cGy (580 cGy/fraction) in the *boost* zone indicated in all cases.
An MD patient with no indication for *boost* was treated with a weekly hypofractionated treatment schedule of 3000 cGy in 5 sessions (600 cGy/fraction) with one fraction per week.

Planning

The planning was carried out in the TPS *PCRT 3D*, version 6.1.1., for an *ONCOR Impression* accelerator *(Siemens Healthineers)* with MLC *OPTIFOCUS* of 82 blades, 1 cm wide in
isocentre. The energy used in all cases was 6 MV. The technique used was 3D-CRT using tangential fields that can include reduced fields or virtual cradles. The dose calculation is performed with a 3 x 3 x 3 x 3

mm grid in each direction using the collapsed cone superposition algorithm described in [39]. The files DVH FILES files analysed by the program are the text files with extension '.grf' that are exported from the planner.

Chapter 4
Results

Data is almost always an imperfect measure of what we are interested in.
- David Spiegelhalter, The Art of Statistics

4.1 Programme checks

It is verified, by analysing the Excel file containing the observables obtained after running the simulation on the 96 patients, that:

- The laterality interpreted was correct in all cases.
- The distance between cuts, Δz, is appropriate in all cases.
- All 384 structures have been successfully identified, for each patient: PTV, ipsilateral lung, heart and contralateral breast.

General operation of the algorithm

Functions have been developed that allow graphs to be made, such as those in figure 3.3, which allow us to corroborate that the algorithm performs the expected processes. The correct generation of the straight line R, of the contour [Haz *(0)]j* and of the pohgons generated in the intersection of the latter with PIp, Cor and MC in several patients of each model, at different angles of incidence *0* and in different cuts *j,* is checked visually by means of these graphs.
In all the cases analysed, the behaviour is as expected.

Volume computation by the programme

For each of the structures of interest for each patient, the relative error between the volume of the structure calculated by the programme (sum of the area of each section of the structure per Az) and the volume of the TPS structure is calculated, according to the following equation:

$$\text{Error relativo } [\%] = 100 \cdot \frac{V_i^{TPS} - V_i^{programa}}{V_i^{TPS}}, \qquad (4.1)$$

where i = PTV, Cor, PIp, MC.

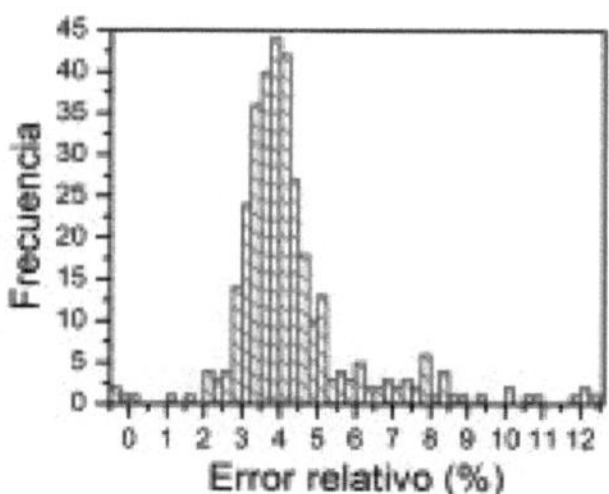

Figure 4.1: Frequency histogram of the relative error between TPS and programme volume.

To analyse the deviation TPS TPS-programme in the computation of the volume of a structure, a frequency histogram of the relative error is presented in Figure 4.1. 4.1.

Interpolation by the programme

The coincidence between the interpolation of the DVH values of the programme with those of the TPS is checked.

4.2 Model calibration

In both models, a correlation line is computed from each OAR is computed for each of the doses between 2.5 and 97.5% of the prescription doses.

Right breast

Figure 4.2 shows the results obtained from the right lung right breast model: Pearson's coefficient r as a function of dose level, linear fits in different ranges of r and values obtained for slope and ordinate at the origin for each dose level.

Left breast

Figures 4.3 and 4.4 show respectively the results of the left breast model obtained for left lung and heart: Pearson's coefficient r as a function of dose level, linear fits in different ranges of r and values obtained for slope and ordinate at the origin for each dose level.

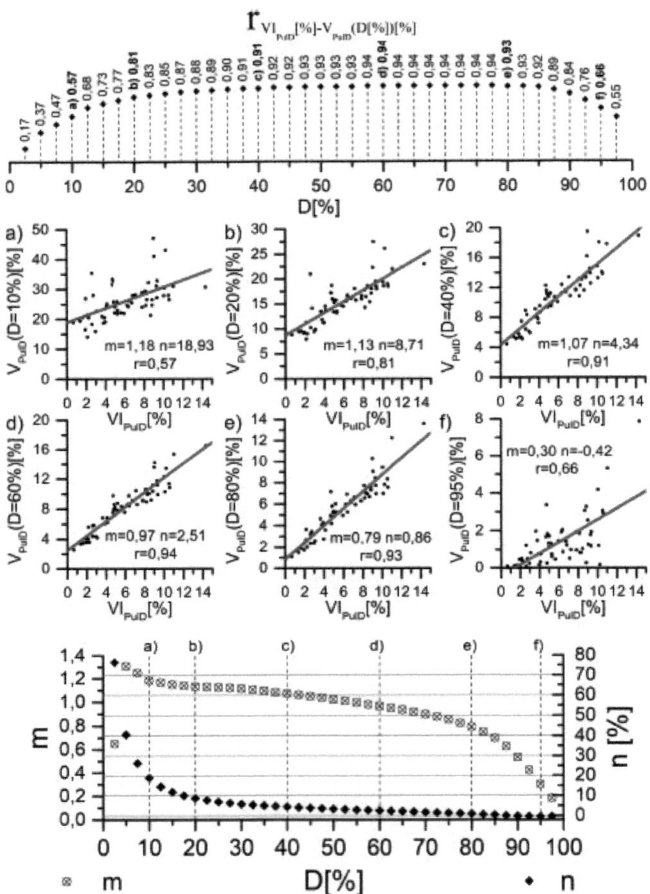

Figura 2: Results for right lung (MD, 59 patients). Top plot: Pearson correlation coefficient between the intersected volume of PulD and the percentage of PulD receiving at least one D dose [%]. Middle graph: Sample fit to the line y = mx + n for D= a) 10%, b) 20%, c) 40%, d) 60%, e) 80%, f) 95%. Bottom plot: slope m and ordinate at the origin n of the line of fit for each dose D [%].

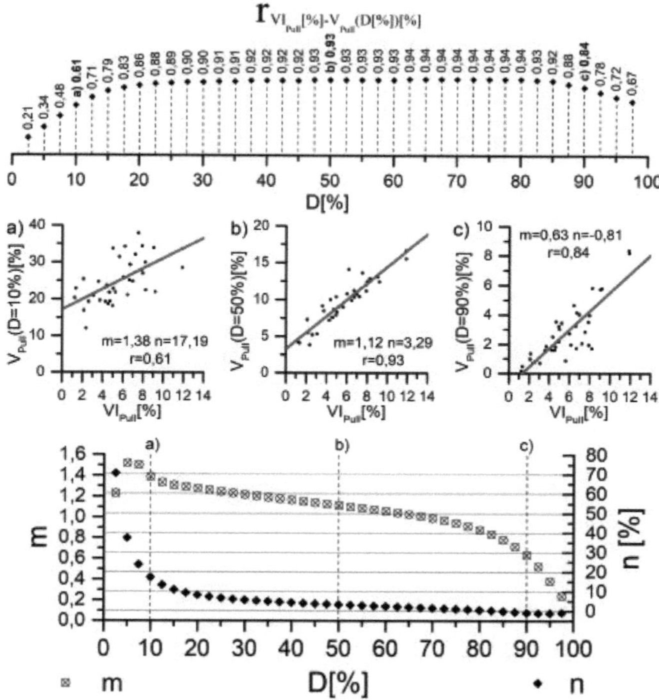

Figura 3: Results for left lung (MI, 37 patients). Top plot: Pearson correlation coefficient between IL lung intersected volume and percentage of IL receiving at least one D dose [%]. Middle graph: Sample fit to the line y = mx + n for D= a) 10%, b) 50%, c) 90%. Bottom graph: slope m and ordinate at the origin n of the line of fit for each dose D [%].

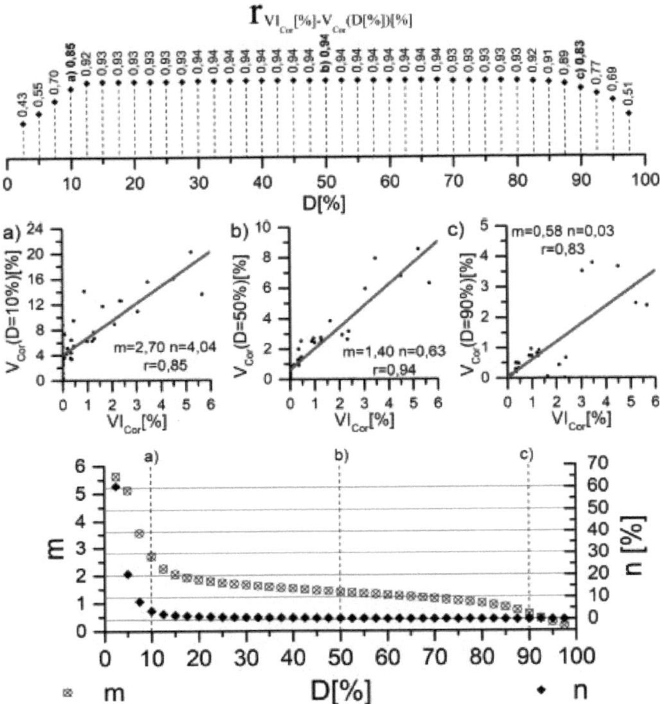

Figura 4: Results for heart (MI, 37 patients). Top plot: Pearson correlation coefficient between Cor intersected volume and percentage of Cor receiving at least one D dose [%]. Middle graph: Sample fit to the line y = mx + n for D= a) 10%, b) 50%, c) 90%. Bottom graph: slope m and ordinate at the origin n of the line of fit for each dose D [%].

Chapter 5
Discussion

Your assumptions are your windows on the world. Scrub them off every once in a while or the light won't come in.

- Alan Alda, *Graduation speech by his daughter*

Volume computation by the programme

The discrepancy in volumes computed by different software from identical structure files is a known and analysed problem in radiotherapy [40]. The DICOM standard defines the coordinates of the structures but leaves the software free to interpret and reconstruct the volumes from them.
The details of the volume calculation method in the TPS are unknown, but are assumed to be more accurate due to, among other possible causes, two related to interpolation of structures.
As can be seen in Figure 4.1, the method for calculating the volume by the programme tends to underestimate the volume with respect to the TPS in most cases. The high frequency of cases around 4 % suggests a systematic component of discrepancy between calculation methods.
The first is the interpolation between axial slices (longitudinal interpolation) implemented by the TPS. The developed program calculates the volume by multiplying the area of the population in a slice by the distance between slices Δz. That is, it assumes that the contour remains constant longitudinally until the next slice (located at a distance of $\Delta z = 5$ mm in most patients), as if it were a prism. However, the TPS are more accurate because they perform interpolations between axial slices. For example, if you contour in one reconstructed axial slice (which cuts the longitudinal axis at zc) and in the next (which cuts the longitudinal axis at en $z_c + \Delta z$),), the TPS would be able to generate contours in axial planes reconstructed between z_c y $z_c + \Delta z$ by interpolation methods. This process would be equivalent in our model to having a shear thickness Δz smaller. If for example $\Delta z = 1$ mm a better match would be expected.
The second reason is the interpolation within the same axial slice. The

developed program, in order to calculate the area of the population that forms the series of points (x,y), joins these coordinates with straight lines (no interpolation). However, the commercial solutions that use the TPS to calculate volumes, perform complex two-dimensional interpolations that join the series of points that define the outline of the structure at each slice with smooth curved lines.
The influence of the systemic component of the relative error on the volume computation is reduced because the final variable, VIOAR[%], is a volume percentage, i.e. a ratio of absolute volumes (intersected by beam and total), both of which are affected by systemic errors and the ratio compensates for them to some extent.
However, some improvement in the correlation results is to be expected if the relative error of the volume computation is reduced.
The large positive dispersion of the relative error of the graph 4.1, reaching values of up to +12.0% in some cases, may be due to structures with a small absolute volume. In these structures the relative error is not a good indicator of accuracy as this value is very sensitive if the measurand is of a similar order of magnitude to the error.

Model results

The results of the linear fit at different doses of the three risk organs show a similar behaviour: The model shows a worse correlation (Pearson's coefficient lower than 0.80) at low doses (lower than 20% of the prescription dose) and very high doses (higher than 90%). At intermediate doses, the Pearson correlation coefficient is always higher than 0.80, being always higher than 0.90 at doses between 35% and 85% of the prescription dose.
This behaviour is in accordance with what is expected from a typical dose distribution in a 3D tangential treatment. Using the case of figure 1.6 b) right as an illustrative support, it can be seen how:

- Lower isodose curves are distributed over larger areas and further away from the PTV than higher isodose curves.
- The isodose curves closest to the prescription dose hardly extend into regions within the organs at risk.

The correlation of the volume enclosed by these isodose surfaces within the organ at risk with the volume of OAR intersected by the tangential beam will be better the greater the spatial overlap of these

two regions.
According to this reasoning, a poorer correlation at low doses is due to the fact that a major part of the volume occupied within the organ at risk lies outside the structure [Haz(0_{opt})|. These zones are not taken into account in the definitions 3.2, 3.3 y 3.4.
At high doses the opposite is the case, but with the same effect. An important part of the volume enclosed by the isodose surfaces close to the prescription dose does fall within the structure [Haz(0_{opt})], but hardly within the organs at risk. Therefore, they also hardly contribute to the magnitudes of the equations 3.2, 3.3 y 3.4.

Other models in the literature

In the literature search, models have been found that predict irradiated volume, under direct beam, of lung only [41] or lung and heart [42]. Another more recent model [43] predicts the mean dose benefit of lung and heart in breast treatments in breath-hold compared to free-breathing. None of them are based on structures but on the correlation between distances measured on the image acquired in the treatment simulation.
The models described in [41] and [42] predict the percentage of lung contained within a tangential bundle from the pulmonary centre distance with a Pearson's coefficient $r=0.89$ in the first article, without distinction according to laterality). In the second article they obtain $r=0.85$ for left lung and $r=0.88$ for right lung, they also correlate this distance with the exposed heart volume, obtaining an $r=0.58$. The volumes predicted in these models are estimators of the degree of exposure of the organ at risk in a tangential treatment, but do not provide information on the doses absorbed.
The values defined in this model according to 3.2, 3.3 and 3.4 and computable from the structures can be good general patient-dependent indicators of the degree of exposure of these organs under the tangential beam.
The third model cited in [43] predicts the mean dose reduction in the heart ($r=0.63$) as a function of the ratio of distances defined in it and the mean dose reduction in the left lung ($r=0.33$) as a function of its free breathing volume.

Limitations of the model

Apart from the limitations in the prediction of the volume of the organ

at risk exposed to low or very high doses, the model presented is restricted to treatments without axillary volume irradiation.
During the construction of the model, right breast patients with affected lymph node volumes were also initially included, however the correlation coefficients obtained were considerably worse because in these cases the VIP ulD does not take into account the over-irradiated lung volume due to the proximity of a lymph node PTV to the lung. As a consequence the model underestimated *VPulD*. The solution in breast cases with irradiated lymph node volumes is not as simple as including in the definition of the beam structure also the PTV because these are not as superficial as the breast and the optimal angle of irradiation of the breast is not the same as that of these volumes. Generally in 3D static treatments, these volumes are irradiated using several fan-shaped beams.
The philosophy of the model makes it suitable for tangential breast treatments where the irradiated volume is superficial and there is a privileged direction of irradiation. These same characteristics make it difficult to extend it to other pathologies or VMAT techniques.
For simplicity, the model presented does not take into account at any time the existence or not of boost. An improvement in results would be expected if a term were included in the *VIOAR* definitions that increases this magnitude inversely proportional to the distance from the boost -OAR contour at each cut.
The execution time of the programme per patient depends mainly and proportionally on the number of cuts where PTV and organs at risk coexist. This number of slices, for the same patient, will be higher if the Az slice thickness is lower. In any case, the simulation time per patient, running the programme on a LENOVO desktop computer with a 2.90 GHz Intel Celeron G4900T processor and obtained from 30 patients, has been less than 20 seconds in all cases, so it is not a limitation.

Assistance in the choice of treatment technique

The model is useful in the choice of treatment technique, predicting whether the volume of OAR exposed to a certain dose is less than that imposed by the constraints before planning the 3D tangential treatment.
The restrictions imposed on each organ at risk are indicated by the prescribing physician on the basis of the fractionation prescribed and

possible particularities of the patient. The models have been created ad hoc in units relative to the prescribed dose in order to be useful for any prescribed prescription. In treatment planning, the aim is not only to comply with the imposed restriction but to obtain an optimal dose distribution, limited by geometrical parameters. This optimal dose distribution in relative values is unique, independent of the prescription. For this reason, it is valid to renormalise each of the DVH curves of the patients treated and thus obtain results with a common coverage criterion in all cases (that 95% of the breast PTV volume is covered by 95% of the prescribed dose) that allows the joint comparison of treatments with different prescriptions as well as with the same prescription but different coverage achieved.

The general process of the prediction consists of exporting the DICOM file of planner structures, running the program on this file to obtain the VI_{OAR}[%] and calculating the VOAR(D) prediction obtained according to the equation 3.1 and the m(D) and n(D) data from the model calibration, in our case, figures: 4.2, 4.3 or 4.4 as appropriate.

The prediction compares VOAR(D) with the restriction imposed by the radiation oncologist, some of which are shown in table 1.1 for patients without cardiac or respiratory comorbidities.

If the predicted volume is less than the imposed restriction, satisfactory results will be obtained with 3D-CRT, otherwise it is advisable to plan directly with a more complex technique.

If the prediction supports a 3D treatment technique by constraint compliance, having run the model has also indicated the optimal gantry angle that should be planned for later.

Conclusions

It is a mistake to confound strangeness with mystery.

- Sherlock Holmes, A Study in Scarlet

A theoretical model has been devised and formulated to correlate a patient-dependent geometric parameter with the volume of a risk organ receiving at least a certain dose in static tangential radiotherapy treatments of the breast.

A Python program has been developed and validated that is able to compute the observables of the model based on its rules.

Using this programme, two models have been calibrated for left and right breast irradiation, using a total of 97 patients treated on an ONCOR accelerator and planned in the PCRT 3D TPS, obtaining a good correlation in the dose range between 20 and 90% of the prescribed dose in the affected breast and an exceptionally good correlation between 35 and 85%. No predictive models with such a good correlation have been found in the literature.

The predictions obtained can be used to employ a personalised treatment technique, avoiding possible re-planning.

Bibliography

[1] Hyuna Sung et al. "Global Cancer Statistics 2020: GLOBOCAN Estimates of Incidence and Mortality Worldwide for 36 Cancers in 185 Countries". In: CA: A Cancer Journal for *Clinicians* 71.3 (2021), pp. 209-249. dOi: https://doi.org/10.3322/caac.21660. uri: https://acsjournals.onlinelibrary.wiley.com/doi/abs/10.3322/caac.21660.

[2] Spanish Network of Cancer Registries. Estimates of cancer incidence in Spain in 2021. Report available at: https://redecan.org. Accessed 21-December-2021.

[3] Robert A. Smith et al. " The randomized trials of breast cancer screening: what have we learned?" In: *Radiologic Clinics of North America* 42.5 (2004), pp. 793-806. issn: 0033-8389. doi: https://doi.org/10.1016/j.rcl.2004.06.014. url: https://www.sciencedirect.com/science/article/pii/S0033838904000880.

[4] Bethany L. Niell et al. "Screening for Breast Cancer". In: *Radiologic Clinics of North America* 55.6 (2017), pp. 1145-1162. issn: 0033-8389. doi: https://doi.org/10.1016/j.rcl.2017.06.004. url: https://www.sciencedirect.com/science/article/pii/S0033838917301070.

[5] National Institute of Health and National Cancer Institute of the United States. *Breast Stage Distribution of SEER Incidence Cases, 2009-2018*. Accessed 21-December-2021. url: https://seer.cancer.gov/statfacts/html/breast.html.

[6] Adrienne G. Waks, Eric P. Winer. "Breast Cancer Treatment: A Review. In: *JAMA* 321.3 (Jan. 2019), pp. 288-300. issn: 0098-7484. doi: 10.1001/jama.2018.19323. url: https://doi.org/10.1001/jama.2018.19323.

[7] Peter Hoskin. *External beam therapy*. 3rd ed. Radiotherapy in Practice. London, England: Oxford University Press, May 2019.

[8] Yasuo Yoshioka et al. *Brachytherapy*. en. 1st ed. Singapore, Singapore: Springer, Aug. 2018.

[9] "Effects of radiotherapy and of differences in the extent of surgery for early breast cancer on local recurrence and 15-year survival: an

overview of the randomised trials. In: *The Lancet* 366.9503 (Dec. 2005), pp. 2087-2106. doi: 10.1016/s0140-6736(05)67887-7. url: https://doi.org/10.1016/s0140-6736(05)67887-7.

[10] Harry Bartelink et al. "Whole-breast irradiation with or without a boost for patients treated with breast-conserving surgery for early breast cancer: 20-year follow-up of a randomised phase 3 trial". In: *The Lancet Oncology* 16.1 (2015), pp. 47-56. issn: 1470-2045. doi: https://doi.org/10.1016/S1470-2045(14)71156-8. url: https://www.sciencedirect.com/science/article/article/pii/S14702045141471 1568.

[11] Jessica Crystal, Mark B. Faries. "Sentinel Lymph Node Biopsy". In: *Surgical Oncology Clinics of North America* 29.3 (July 2020), pp. 401-414. doi: 10.1016/j.soc.2020.02.006. url: https://doi.org/10.1016/j.soc.2020.02.006.

[12] Chirag Shah, Zahraa Al-Hilli, Frank Vicini. "Advances in Breast Cancer Radiotherapy: Implications for Current and Future Practice". In: *JCO Oncology Practice* 17.12 (2021), pp. 697-706. doi: 10.1200/OP.21.00635. url: https://doi.org/10.1200/OP.21.00635.

[13] Thalita Monteiro Obal, Neida Maria Patias Volpi, Simone Aparecida Miloca. "Multiob jective approach in plans for treatment of cancer by radiotherapy". In: *Pesquisa Operacional* 33.2 (Aug. 2013), pp. 269-282. doi: 10.1590/s010101-74382013000200008. url: https://doi. org/10.1590/s010101-74382013000200008.

[14] Zoltan Varga et al. "Radiation dose to the nodal regions during prone versus supine breast irradiation". In: *Therapeutics and Clinical Risk Management* (May 2014), p. 367. dOi: 10.2147/tcrm.s59483. url: https://doi.org/10.2147/tcrm.s59483.

[15] Semaya Natalia Chen, Prabhakar Ramachandran, Pradip Deb. "Dosimetric comparative study of 3DCRT, IMRT, VMAT, Ecomp, and Hybrid techniques for breast radiation therapy". In: *Radiation Oncology Journal* 38.4 (Dec. 2020), pp. 270-281. dOi: 10.3857/roj.2020.00619. url:

https://doi.org/10.3857/roj.2020.00619.

[16] International DICOM standard website: https://www.dicomstandard.org/. Accessed 28-Jan-2022.

[17] Pieter Deseyne et al. "Whole breast and regional nodal irradiation in prone versus supine position in left sided breast cancer". In: *Radiation Oncology* 12.1 (May 2017). dOi: 10.1186/ s13014-017-0828-6. url: https://doi.org/10.1186/s13014-017-0828-6.

[18] Vincent Vakaet et al. "5-Year Outcomes of a Randomized Trial Comparing Prone and Supine Whole Breast Irradiation in Large-Breasted Women". In: *International Journal of Radiation Oncology-Biology-Physics* 110.3 (July 2021), pp. 766-771. dOi: 10.1016/j.ijrobp.2021. 01.026. url: https://doi.org/10.1016/j.ijrobp.2021.01.026.

[19] Carmen Bergom et al. "Deep Inspiration Breath Hold: Techniques and Advantages for Cardiac Sparing During Breast Cancer Irradiation". In: *Frontiers in Oncology* 8 (2018), p. 87. issn: 2234-943X. dOi: 10.3389/fonc.2018.00087. url: https://www.frontiersin.org/ article/10.3389/fonc.2018.00087.

[20] Xinzhuo Wang et al. "Is prone free breathing better than supine deep inspiration breathhold for left whole-breast radiotherapy? A dosimetric analysis". In: *Strahlentherapie und Onkologie* 197.4 (Jan. 2021), pp. 317-331. dOi: 10 . 1007/s00066-020-01731-8. url: https://doi.org/10.1007/s00066-020-01731-8.

[21] Delia Ciardo et al. "Atlas-based segmentation in breast cancer radiotherapy: Evaluation of specific and generic-purpose atlases". In: *The Breast* 32 (Apr. 2017), pp. 44-52. dOi: 10. 1016/j.breast.2016.12.010. url: https://doi.org/10.1016/j.breast.2016.12.010.

[22] Nalee Kim et al. "Atlas-based auto-segmentation for postoperative radiotherapy planning in endometrial and cervical cancers". In: *Radiation Oncology* 15.1 (May 2020). dOi: 10.1186/ s13014-020-01562-y. url: https://doi.org/10.1186/s13014-020-01562-y.

[23] Timo Kiljunen et al. "A Deep Learning-Based Automated CT Segmentation of Prostate Cancer Anatomy for Radiation Therapy Planning-A Retrospective Multicenter Study". In: *Diagnostics* 10.11

(Nov. 2020), p. 959. dOi: 10.3390/diagnostics10110959. url: https: //doi.org/10.3390/diagnostics10110959.

[24] *International Commission on Radiation Units and Measurements Report 62: Prescribing, Recording and Reporting Photon Beam Therapy.*

[25] Joanne S Haviland et al. "The UK Standardisation of Breast Radiotherapy (START) trials of radiotherapy hypofractionation for treatment of early breast cancer: 10-year follow-up results of two randomised controlled trials". In: *Lancet Oncol.* 14.11 (Oct. 2013), pp. 1086-1094.

[26] Adrian Murray Brunt et al. " Ten-Year Results of FAST: A Randomized Controlled Trial of 5-Fraction Whole-Breast Radiotherapy for Early Breast Cancer". In: *Journal of Clinical Oncology* 38.28 (2020), pp. 3261-3272. dOi: 10.1200/JCO.19.02750. url: https://doi. org/10.1200/JCO.19.02750.

[27] Adrian Murray Brunt et al. "Hypofractionated breast radiotherapy for 1 week versus 3 weeks (FAST-Forward): 5-year efficacy and late normal tissue effects results from a multicentre, non-inferiority, randomised, phase 3 trial". In: *The Lancet* 395.10237 (May 2020), pp. 16131626. dOi: 10.1016/s0140-6736(20)30932-6. url: https://doi.org/10.1016/s0140- 6736(20)30932-6.

[28] Sasa Mutic et al. " Quality assurance for computed-tomography simulators and the computed- tomography-simulation process: Report of the AAPM Radiation Therapy Committee Task Group No. 66". In: *Medical Physics* 30.10 (Sept. 2003), pp. 2762-2792. dOi: 10.1118/1. 1609271. url: https://doi.org/10.1118/1.1609271.

[29] Jennifer B. Smilowitz et al. Smilowitz et al. "AAPM Medical Physics Practice Guideline 5.a.: Commissioning and QA of Treatment Planning Dose Calculations - Megavoltage Photon and Electron Beams". In: *Journal of Applied Clinical Medical Physics* 16.5 (2015), pp. 14-34. dOi: https : / /doi . org/ 10 . 1120 / jacmp . v16i5 . 5768. url: https : // aapm . onlinelibrary . wiley.com/doi/abs/10.1120/jacmp.v16i5.5768.

[30] Eric E. Klein et al. "Task Group 142 report: Quality assurance of medical accelerators)". In: *Medical Physics* 36.9Part1 (Aug. 2009),

pp. 4197-4212. doi: 10.1118/1.3190392. url: https://doi.org/10.1118/1.3190392.

[31] Indra J. Das et al. "Accelerator beam data commissioning equipment and procedures: Report of the TG-106 of the Therapy Physics Committee of the AAPM". In: *Medical Physics* 35.9 (Aug. 2008), pp. 4186-4215. doi: 10.1118/1.2969070. url: https://doi.org/10.1118/ 1.2969070.

[32] Seung Yong Song et al. "Hypofractionated Radiotherapy With Volumetric Modulated Arc Therapy Decreases Postoperative Complications in Prosthetic Breast Reconstructions: A Clinicopathologic Study". In: *Frontiers in Oncology* 10 (2020), p. 2526. issn: 2234-943X. doi: 10 . 3389 / fonc . 2020 . 577136. url: https : / /www . frontiersin . org / article / 10 . 3389/fonc.2020.577136.

[33] Javier Sanz et al. " Once-Weekly Hypofractionated Radiotherapy for Breast Cancer in Elderly Patients: Efficacy and Tolerance in 486 Patients". In: *BioMed Research International* 2018 (2018), pp. 1-9. doi: 10.1155/2018/8321871. url: https://doi.org/10.1155/2018/ 8321871.

[34] Raquel Ciervide et al. "Neoadjuvant Chemoradiation for Unfavourable BreastCancer Patients: A Prospective Cohort Study". In: *Journal of Clinical Trials* 9:3 (2019).

[35] Wei Zhang et al. "Dosimetry and Feasibility Studies of Volumetric Modulated Arc Therapy With Deep Inspiration Breath-Hold Using Optical Surface Management System for Left-Sided Breast Cancer Patients". In: *Frontiers in Oncology* 10 (2020), p. 1711. issn: 2234-943X. doi: 10.3389/fonc.2020.01711. url: https://www.frontiersin.org/article/10.3389/ fonc.2020.01711.

[36] Moyed Miften et al. " Tolerance limits and methodologies for IMRT measurement-based verification QA: Recommendations of AAPM Task Group No. 218". In: *Medical Physics* 45.4 (Mar. 2018), e53-e83. doi: 10.1002/mp.12810. url: https://doi.org/10.1002/mp.12810.

[37] Birgitte V. Offersen et al. "ESTRO consensus guideline on target volume delineation for elective radiation therapy of early stage breast cancer". In: *Radiotherapy and Oncology* 114.1 (2015), pp. 3-10. issn:

0167-8140. doi: https://doi.org/10.1016/j.radonc.2014.11.030. url: https://www.sciencedirect.com/science/article/pii/S016781401400 5246.

[38] Benjamin D. Smith et al. "Radiation therapy for the whole breast: Executive summary of an American Society for Radiation Oncology (ASTRO) evidence-based guideline". In: *Practical Radiation Oncology* 8.3 (May 2018), pp. 145-152. doi: 10.1016/j .prro.2018.01.012. url: https://doi.org/10.1016/j.prro.2018.01.012.

[39] Alejandro Garrna Romero, Miguel Canellas Anoz, Dolores Lardies Fleta. "Development and Monte Carlo verification of a collapsed cone superposition algorithm for the calculation of photon beams in radiotherapy". In: *Rev. Med.* 10 (Nov. 2009), pp. 187-198.

[40] Richa Sharma et al. "A Statistical Study based on comparison between two treatment planning systems while exporting RT structure set". In: (2015), pp. 364-367. doi: 10.1007/978-3- 319-19387-8_87. url: https://doi.org/10.1007/978-3-319-19387-8_87.

[41] Bruce A. Bornstein et al. " Can simulation measurements be used to predict the irradiated lung volume in the tangential fields in patients treated for breast cancer?" In: *International Journal of Radiation Oncology, Biology, Physics* 18.1 (Jan. 1990), pp. 181-187. doi: 10.1016/0360- 3016(90)90282-o. url: https://doi.org/10.1016/0360-3016(90)90282-o.

[42] Indra J Das et al. "Lung and heart dose volume analyses with CT simulator in radiation treatment of breast cancer". In: *International Journal of Radiation Oncology, Biology, Physics* 42.1 (Aug. 1998), pp. 11-19. doi: 10 . 1016 / s0360 - 3016(98) 00200 - 4. url: https : //doi.org/10.1016/s0360-3016(98)00200-4.

[43] Ning Cao et al. "Predictors of cardiac and lung dose sparing in DIBH for left breast treatment".
In: *Physica Medica 67* (Nov. 2019), pp. 27-33. dOi: 10.1016/j.ejmp.2019.09.240. uri: https://doi.org/10.1016/j.ejmp.2019.09.240.

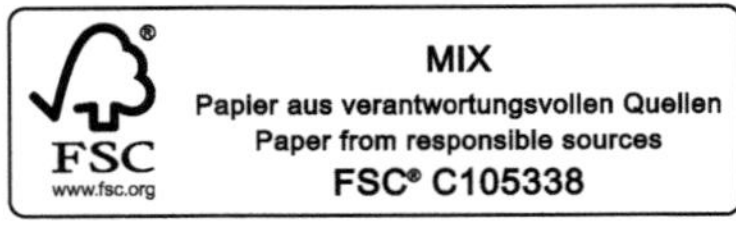

Printed by Books on Demand GmbH, Norderstedt / Germany